THRIVING WITH HISTAMINE INTOLERANCE

Understanding Symptoms,Diagnosis,Diet Plans and Effective Treatments/Management Strategies

Dr Jude Hills

Table of Contents

What to Expect

Welcome to "Thriving with Histamine Intolerance," a comprehensive guide designed to help you understand, manage, and thrive despite the challenges posed by histamine intolerance. This book aims to empower you with knowledge and practical strategies, providing you with the tools necessary to live a healthy, balanced life.

Understanding Histamine Intolerance

Histamine intolerance can be perplexing and frustrating, but understanding its mechanisms is the first step toward effective management. In the initial chapters, we'll delve into the science behind histamine intolerance, exploring what histamine is, how it functions in the body, and what happens when its levels become unbalanced. You'll learn about the role of diamine oxidase (DAO), the enzyme responsible for breaking down histamine, and why a deficiency or malfunction of DAO can lead to symptoms ranging from headaches and digestive issues to skin reactions and respiratory problems.

Treatment and Management Options

Managing histamine intolerance requires a multifaceted approach. We'll cover:

Dietary Modifications

Diet is the cornerstone of managing histamine intolerance. We'll provide a detailed overview of a low-histamine diet, including:

- Foods to Avoid: Learn about high-histamine foods and histamine liberators that can trigger your symptoms.
- Foods to Include: Discover safe food options that are low in histamine and rich in nutrients.

Supplements and Medications

While diet plays a crucial role, supplements and medications can also support your management plan:

- DAO Supplements: Understand how these supplements can help break down histamine in your digestive tract.
- Vitamins and Minerals: Explore how vitamin C, vitamin B6, magnesium, and quercetin can aid in managing histamine levels.
- Medications: Learn about antihistamines and other medications that can help control your symptoms when dietary adjustments alone aren't enough.

Recovery Journey

Recovering from histamine intolerance is a journey that requires patience and persistence. We'll guide you through:

Timeline of Recovery

- Short-Term vs. Long-Term Expectations: Understand what improvements to expect in the short term and how to maintain progress in the long term.

Monitoring Progress

- Keeping a Symptom and Food Diary: Learn how to track your symptoms and food intake to identify triggers and monitor improvements.
- Regular Medical Check-Ups: Discover the importance of ongoing medical supervision and adjustments to your management plan.

Diet Planning and Recipes

Crafting a diet plan can be overwhelming, but we're here to help:

Foods to Avoid and Include

- High-Histamine Foods: Detailed lists of foods
to steer clear of to avoid triggering symptoms.
- Low-Histamine Foods: Extensive lists of safe
food options that are nutritious and delicious.

Meal Planning Tips

- Creating Balanced Meals: Tips on how to
create balanced, nutritious meals that adhere to
a low-histamine diet.
- Sample Meal Plans: Example meal plans to
help you get started on your journey.

Recipes

Enjoy a variety of recipes tailored to a
low-histamine diet:

- Breakfast: Start your day with healthy,
low-histamine breakfast options.

- Lunch and Dinner: Find inspiration for satisfying and delicious main meals.
- Snacks: Discover snack ideas that will keep you energized throughout the day.

Long-Term Management and Living with Histamine Intolerance

Living with histamine intolerance requires ongoing adjustments and support. We'll cover:

Monitoring and Adjusting Diet and Lifestyle

- Adapting to Changes in Tolerance: How to recognize and respond to changes in your tolerance levels over time.

Psychological and Emotional Support

- Coping Strategies: Practical strategies to help you manage the emotional and psychological aspects of histamine intolerance.
- Support Groups and Resources: Information on where to find support and connect with

others who understand what you're going through.

Tips for Eating Out

- Managing Histamine Intolerance in Social Situations and Restaurants: Strategies for dining out and socializing without compromising your health.

Future Directions in Research

We'll look at the horizon for histamine intolerance management:

Emerging Treatments and Diagnostic Tools

- New Therapies: Insight into promising new treatments and supplements that are being developed.
- Advanced Diagnostics: Information on cutting-edge diagnostic tools that could revolutionize the way histamine intolerance is diagnosed and managed.

Conclusion

In our final chapter, we'll summarize key points and reflect on the journey of living with histamine intolerance. We'll also look to the future, highlighting ongoing research and emerging treatments that offer hope for improved management and quality of life.

"Thriving with Histamine Intolerance" is more than just a guide; it's a companion on your journey toward better health and well-being. By the end of this book, you will have a deeper understanding of your condition, a solid plan for managing your symptoms, and the confidence to live a full, vibrant life despite histamine intolerance. Let's embark on this journey together, equipped with knowledge, strategies, and the support you need to thrive.

INTRODUCTION

Imagine enjoying a plate of aged cheese and a glass of red wine, only to find yourself experiencing an unexpected headache or skin rash shortly after. These could be symptoms of histamine intolerance, a condition that's not widely recognized but can significantly impact daily life. As more people become aware of this condition, it's essential to understand what histamine intolerance is, how prevalent it is, and why it matters. This article aims to delve into these aspects, providing a comprehensive overview of histamine intolerance.

Overview of Histamine Intolerance

Definition

Histamine intolerance is a condition where the body is unable to break down histamine efficiently, leading to an accumulation that causes various symptoms. Histamine is a naturally occurring compound involved in local immune responses, regulating physiological functions in the gut, and acting as a neurotransmitter. It is found in many foods and is also released by the body during allergic reactions. Normally, the enzyme diamine oxidase (DAO) breaks down histamine in the digestive tract. However, in individuals with histamine intolerance, this process is impaired, leading to symptoms such as headaches, skin rashes, digestive issues, and respiratory problems.

Prevalence and Demographic Insights

While histamine intolerance is often underdiagnosed due to its varied and nonspecific symptoms, it is estimated that around 1-3% of the population may be affected. This condition seems to be more common in middle-aged adults, particularly women, who are often more sensitive to fluctuations in hormones that can affect histamine levels. Additionally, individuals with gastrointestinal disorders like irritable bowel syndrome (IBS) or those taking certain medications that inhibit DAO activity are at higher risk. Despite its prevalence, many people remain unaware of histamine intolerance, mistaking it for allergies or other conditions.

Importance of Understanding Histamine Intolerance

Understanding histamine intolerance is crucial for several reasons. First, it can significantly improve the quality of life for those affected. Identifying and managing histamine intolerance through dietary adjustments and lifestyle changes can alleviate chronic symptoms that are often misattributed to other causes. Second, increased awareness among healthcare providers can lead to better diagnosis and treatment plans, reducing the trial-and-error period that many patients endure. Lastly, understanding the condition can promote further research into its mechanisms and potential therapies, offering hope for more effective solutions in the future.

An Engaging and Informative Exploration

Histamine intolerance, though not widely recognized, is a fascinating condition that underscores the complexity of our body's interactions with the foods we consume and the substances we produce. Imagine your body as a highly efficient factory, where every process is meticulously timed and executed. In the case of histamine intolerance, one of these processes – the breakdown of histamine – is compromised, leading to an overflow of histamine that the body can't manage.

Let's consider the impact of this on everyday life. Picture this: you're at a dinner party, enjoying a delightful array of cheese, cured meats, and perhaps a bit of red wine. These foods are notorious for their high histamine content. For most people, the body processes these histamines without any issues. However, for someone with histamine intolerance, this indulgence can quickly turn into a nightmare of migraines, hives, or digestive discomfort.

Histamine intolerance doesn't discriminate, but it does show a preference for certain demographics. Middle-aged women, for instance, often find themselves more susceptible, possibly due to hormonal changes that affect histamine metabolism. Moreover, those with gastrointestinal disorders are at an added disadvantage, as their already compromised digestive systems struggle even more with histamine breakdown.

Recognizing histamine intolerance can be a game-changer. Imagine suffering from chronic headaches and sinus issues for years, only to discover that the culprit isn't pollen or stress, but the aged cheese and glass of wine you enjoy so much. By identifying the root cause, individuals can make informed choices about their diets and lifestyles, leading to significant improvements in their overall well-being.

As awareness of histamine intolerance grows, so does the potential for better medical guidance and support. Currently, many patients endure a lengthy and frustrating journey of misdiagnosis, often undergoing numerous tests and treatments that provide little relief. Increased understanding and recognition of histamine intolerance can shorten this journey, providing quicker, more effective solutions.

Research into histamine intolerance is still in its infancy, but the potential benefits are immense. As scientists delve deeper into the mechanisms behind this condition, they could uncover new treatments that go beyond simple dietary restrictions. Imagine a world where a simple supplement or medication could regulate histamine levels, allowing individuals to enjoy their favorite foods without fear of debilitating symptoms.

Histamine intolerance is a condition that deserves more attention and understanding. By exploring its definition, prevalence, and the importance of awareness, we can better appreciate the impact it has on those affected. As we continue to learn and share knowledge about histamine intolerance, we can hope for a future where its management is straightforward and effective, transforming the lives of many who suffer in silence. So, the next time you enjoy a plate of cheese or a glass of wine, spare a thought for the hidden complexities within our bodies and the importance of understanding conditions like histamine intolerance.

CHAPTER ONE

Histamine and Its Role in the Body

Histamine is a term that might ring a bell if you've ever dealt with allergies, but its role in the body is much more nuanced and fascinating than just being the culprit behind a runny nose or itchy eyes. This chapter delves into the multifaceted world of histamine, exploring its chemical structure, functions, and sources, both from within our bodies and from the foods we eat.

1.1 What is Histamine?

Chemical Structure and Function

At its core, histamine is a simple molecule, but don't let its simplicity fool you. Chemically, histamine is an amine derived from the amino acid histidine. It consists of an imidazole ring attached to an ethylamine chain, making it a small but potent biochemical messenger with the chemical formula $C_5H_9N_3$.

Histamine's function is diverse and critical. It's involved in several key processes in the body, acting as a neurotransmitter in the brain, regulating gut function, and playing a pivotal role in the immune response. When you think of histamine, imagine it as a versatile actor in a complex drama, taking on different roles depending on the scene.

Role in the Immune System

Histamine's most well-known role is in the immune system, where it acts as a first responder to invaders. When your body encounters allergens like pollen or pet dander, certain immune cells, called mast cells and basophils, release histamine. This release triggers a cascade of events designed to expel the intruder. Blood vessels dilate, causing redness and swelling, while increased permeability allows immune cells to reach the site of infection or irritation more easily.

This inflammatory response, while uncomfortable, is a crucial part of your body's defense mechanism. However, in cases of histamine intolerance or allergies, this response can be excessive, leading to symptoms like hives, itching, and difficulty breathing.

Histamine Metabolism

To prevent histamine levels from running amok, your body relies on three key enzymes: histamine-N-methyltransferase (HNMT), diamine oxidase (DAO), and monoamine oxidase (MAO). These enzymes are like diligent janitors, cleaning up excess histamine to maintain balance.

Histamine-N-methyltransferase (HNMT) is primarily active in the central nervous system and liver, where it inactivates histamine by methylation. This process involves transferring a methyl group to the histamine molecule, rendering it inactive.

Diamine oxidase (DAO), on the other hand, is crucial for breaking down histamine in the digestive tract. DAO degrades histamine by oxidative deamination, converting it into imidazole acetaldehyde, which is then further metabolized and excreted. DAO concentrations are particularly high in the intestines and placenta. When DAO activity is compromised, whether due to genetic factors, certain medications, or gut issues, histamine can accumulate, leading to the symptoms associated with histamine intolerance.

1.2 SOURCES OF HISTAMINE

Endogenous Production

Histamine is produced endogenously in various tissues throughout the body. It is stored in high concentrations within mast cells and basophils, ready to be released during an immune response. The brain also synthesizes histamine, where it functions as a neurotransmitter, influencing wakefulness, appetite, and cognitive processes.

The body's production of histamine is a finely tuned process, essential for maintaining homeostasis. For example, in the brain, histamine helps regulate the sleep-wake cycle by promoting wakefulness during the day. In the stomach, histamine stimulates the release of gastric acid, aiding in digestion. Enterochromaffin-like cells (ECL cells) in the stomach and intestines are significant sources of non-mast cell histamine.

Exogenous Sources

While your body produces histamine, it also comes from external sources, primarily through diet. Understanding these exogenous sources is crucial for managing histamine levels, especially for those with histamine intolerance.

Foods and Drinks

Histamine is naturally present in various foods, particularly those that are aged, fermented, or processed. Think of foods like aged cheeses, cured meats, and fermented products such as sauerkraut and soy sauce. These foods contain high levels of histamine because of bacterial action during fermentation and aging.

Alcoholic beverages, especially red wine and beer, are also significant sources of histamine. The fermentation process involved in making these drinks leads to histamine accumulation. For some, a glass of wine might be an enjoyable end to the day, but for those sensitive to histamine, it could mean a night of headaches and discomfort.

Certain foods can also prompt the body to release histamine. These include citrus fruits, strawberries, tomatoes, nuts, and chocolate. While these foods might not contain high levels of histamine themselves, they can trigger the release of histamine stored in your body's cells.

To add to the complexity, some foods block the action of DAO, the enzyme responsible for breaking down histamine. Alcohol, energy drinks, and black tea can inhibit DAO, leading to higher histamine levels in the body. This interaction explains why some people might feel particularly unwell after consuming certain foods and drinks.

An Engaging and Informative Exploration

Histamine is like an unsung hero with a tricky reputation. Its involvement in critical bodily functions contrasts sharply with its role in causing allergic reactions and intolerance symptoms. Understanding histamine means recognizing its dual nature: indispensable for health yet potentially disruptive when out of balance.

Imagine histamine as the conductor of an orchestra. When everything is in harmony, histamine ensures that the body's systems work together seamlessly, responding to threats and regulating vital functions. But if one section starts playing too loudly or out of sync, the entire performance suffers, leading to the cacophony of symptoms associated with histamine intolerance.

Managing histamine intolerance often requires becoming a detective of your own body, identifying which foods and drinks trigger symptoms and making informed choices to maintain balance. It's a journey of self-discovery and adaptation, but with knowledge and awareness, it becomes possible to enjoy life without the constant interference of histamine-related issues.

Histamine is a fascinating and multifaceted molecule that plays a critical role in our bodies. From its chemical structure to its functions in the immune system and beyond, understanding histamine provides insight into how our bodies maintain balance and respond to external challenges. By recognizing the sources of histamine, both endogenous and exogenous, we can better manage our health and wellbeing. As you continue to explore the world of histamine, remember that this small molecule holds the key to many of the body's essential processes, making it a vital, if sometimes troublesome, component of our biological symphony.

CHAPTER TWO

Symptoms of Histamine Intolerance

Histamine intolerance, a condition resulting from an imbalance between the body's stored histamine and its ability to degrade it, can manifest in a variety of ways. Histamine is a biogenic amine present in numerous foods, and its accumulation can lead to a range of symptoms resembling allergic reactions. This chapter delves into the diverse and complex symptoms associated with histamine intolerance, examining both common and less common manifestations, and includes real-life patient stories to illustrate these experiences.

2.1 Common Symptoms

Histamine intolerance affects various bodily systems, with symptoms often overlapping with those of other conditions, making it challenging to diagnose.

Gastrointestinal Issues

The gastrointestinal (GI) tract is one of the most affected areas, with patients frequently experiencing:

- **Bloating:** This uncomfortable sensation of fullness and tightness in the abdomen is often due to excess gas or fluid accumulation, which is likely a result of histamine's role in increasing intestinal permeability and causing inflammation.

- **Diarrhea:** Frequent, loose, or watery bowel movements are common. Histamine can increase intestinal motility, speeding up the transit of food and leading to diarrhea, which can be particularly disruptive and cause dehydration and nutrient deficiencies if chronic.

- **Stomach Pain:** Cramping or discomfort in the abdominal area is another frequent complaint. Histamine influences the production of stomach acid, and excessive histamine can lead to hyperacidity, causing stomach pain and even ulcers in severe cases.

Dermatological Symptoms

The impact of histamine on the skin is highly visible and often distressing. These symptoms tend to flare up after consuming high-histamine foods or exposure to allergens.

- **Hives:** Raised, red, itchy welts appear on the skin as a classic allergic reaction caused by histamine release from mast cells, leading to swelling and itchiness.

- **Itching:** Persistent itchiness without visible hives can affect any part of the body and is often exacerbated by heat, stress, or certain foods.

- **Flushing:** Sudden redness and warmth, usually on the face and neck, occurs when histamine causes the blood vessels to dilate, increasing blood flow to the skin's surface.

Respiratory Symptoms

Histamine can also affect the respiratory system, causing symptoms similar to allergic reactions or respiratory infections.

- **Nasal Congestion:** A stuffy or blocked nose results from histamine causing the blood vessels in the nasal passages to swell, making it difficult to breathe through the nose.

- **Asthma-like Symptoms:** Wheezing, coughing, and shortness of breath can occur as histamine causes bronchoconstriction, narrowing the airways and leading to symptoms similar to asthma.

Neurological Symptoms

As a neurotransmitter, histamine can significantly affect the nervous system, contributing to various neurological symptoms.

- **Headaches:** Particularly migraines. High histamine levels can dilate blood vessels in the brain, leading to painful headaches. Many individuals with histamine intolerance report frequent and severe migraines.

- **Dizziness:** A sensation of spinning or light-headedness can occur as histamine affects the inner ear and balance mechanisms.

Cardiovascular Symptoms

Histamine's influence extends to the cardiovascular system, causing symptoms that can be alarming and uncomfortable.

- **Hypotension**: Low blood pressure results from histamine-induced vasodilation, which can lead to dizziness, fainting, or light-headedness.

- **Tachycardia:** An abnormally fast heart rate occurs as the heart beats faster in response to a drop in blood pressure, causing palpitations and a racing heart.

2.2 Less Common Symptoms

Histamine intolerance can also present with less common symptoms that are frequently overlooked or misattributed to other conditions.

Musculoskeletal Pain

Some individuals experience pain in their muscles and joints due to histamine-induced inflammation in the musculoskeletal system.

- **Arthralgia:** Joint pain without swelling, often described as aching or stiffness.

- **Myalgia:** Muscle pain, ranging from mild discomfort to severe, debilitating pain.

Menstrual Irregularities

Histamine can influence hormonal balance and reproductive health, leading to:

- **Irregular Menstrual Cycles:** Variations in the length and intensity of menstrual periods. Women with histamine intolerance may experience more frequent, heavy, or painful periods.

- **Premenstrual Symptoms:** Increased severity of premenstrual syndrome (PMS) symptoms, such as mood swings, bloating, and breast tenderness.

Chronic Fatigue

Many people with histamine intolerance report feeling persistently tired, regardless of how much rest they get. This chronic fatigue can be overwhelming and is often accompanied by other symptoms such as brain fog, difficulty concentrating, and overall low energy levels.

2.3 Case Studies and Patient Stories

To better understand the real-life impact of histamine intolerance, let's look at a few case studies and patient stories.

Case Study 1: Emma's Digestive Dilemma

Emma, a 34-year-old teacher, had been suffering from bloating and diarrhea for years. Despite numerous tests and dietary changes, her symptoms persisted. It wasn't until she saw a specialist in food intolerances that she was diagnosed with histamine intolerance. By identifying and avoiding high-histamine foods like aged cheese and red wine, Emma saw a significant reduction in her symptoms, allowing her to lead a more comfortable and active life.

Case Study 2: David's Dermatological Distress

David, a 42-year-old accountant, frequently broke out in hives and experienced severe itching, especially after meals. His condition was misdiagnosed as eczema until a detailed food diary and subsequent testing revealed a histamine intolerance. With a new diet plan and the use of antihistamines, David's skin condition improved drastically, and he could enjoy social meals without fear of flare-ups.

Case Study 3: Sophie's Respiratory Relief

Sophie, a 28-year-old athlete, often found herself short of breath and wheezing after consuming certain foods. Initially thought to be exercise-induced asthma, further investigation uncovered that her symptoms correlated with high-histamine foods. Adjusting her diet allowed Sophie to manage her symptoms effectively and continue her training without respiratory distress.

Case Study 4: Mark's Mysterious Migraines

Mark, a 50-year-old engineer, suffered from debilitating migraines that impacted his work and personal life. Multiple treatments failed to provide relief until he discovered the link between his diet and histamine intolerance. By eliminating trigger foods like processed meats and fermented products, Mark significantly reduced the frequency and intensity of his migraines, improving his overall quality of life.

Histamine intolerance presents a wide spectrum of symptoms, affecting various bodily systems. Understanding these symptoms and their underlying mechanisms is crucial for managing the condition effectively. Through awareness, proper diagnosis, and dietary management, individuals with histamine intolerance can find relief and lead healthier, more comfortable lives. The patient stories highlighted in this chapter underscore the importance of personalized approaches to identify and mitigate triggers, offering hope and strategies for those navigating the complexities of histamine intolerance.

CHAPTER THREE

Diagnosis of Histamine Intolerance

Histamine intolerance is a multifaceted condition that manifests with a diverse range of symptoms, often overlapping with other health issues. The diagnostic process for histamine intolerance is intricate, requiring a blend of medical history evaluation, symptom assessment, dietary interventions, blood tests, and differential diagnosis to accurately identify and manage the condition.

3.1 Medical History and Symptom Assessment

Importance of Tracking Symptoms and Dietary Habits

The first step in diagnosing histamine intolerance involves a thorough review of the patient's medical history and detailed symptom assessment. Given the varied nature of histamine intolerance symptoms, careful documentation is essential.

Tracking Symptoms:
- Patients should maintain a detailed symptom diary, recording the onset, duration, and intensity of their symptoms. Common

symptoms to track include gastrointestinal issues (such as bloating, diarrhea, and stomach pain), skin reactions (like hives and itching), respiratory difficulties (nasal congestion and asthma-like symptoms), neurological issues (headaches and dizziness), and cardiovascular symptoms (tachycardia and low blood pressure).
- This documentation helps identify patterns or specific triggers related to histamine-rich foods, environmental changes, or stress levels.

Monitoring Dietary Habits:
- A comprehensive food diary is equally important. Patients should log all food and beverage intake, including meal times, snacks, supplements, and medications.
- Identifying the correlation between food consumption and symptom onset can provide critical clues. Certain foods, such as aged cheeses, processed meats, fermented products, and alcohol, are known high-histamine triggers.
- By cross-referencing food intake with symptom occurrence, healthcare providers can

better pinpoint potential histamine intolerance and differentiate it from other dietary-related issues.

3.2 Elimination Diet

An elimination diet is a practical method for identifying histamine intolerance, involving the systematic removal and gradual reintroduction of high-histamine foods to observe changes in symptoms.

Steps to Implement an Elimination Diet

1. Preparation:
   - Before starting the elimination diet, patients should consult a healthcare provider or dietitian to ensure their nutritional needs are met.
   - Preparation includes identifying foods high in histamine and planning alternative meals that exclude these items.

2. Elimination Phase:

- During this phase, patients eliminate all high-histamine foods from their diet for 2-4 weeks. High-histamine foods include aged cheeses, cured meats, alcohol, fermented foods, certain fish, and some fruits and vegetables like tomatoes and spinach.

- It is also essential to avoid other potential triggers such as alcohol and medications that either release histamine or inhibit its breakdown.

3. Monitoring:

- Throughout the elimination phase, patients should continue documenting their symptoms and dietary intake. This ongoing monitoring helps determine if symptom improvement correlates with dietary changes.

Reintroduction Phase

1. Gradual Reintroduction:

- After the elimination phase, patients gradually reintroduce high-histamine foods one at a time, typically every 3-5 days, while monitoring for any return of symptoms.

- This method helps identify specific food triggers, providing clear evidence of histamine intolerance.

2. Evaluation:

- If symptoms reoccur during the reintroduction phase, the offending food should be eliminated again. Patients should wait for symptoms to resolve before reintroducing another food.

- Detailed records during this phase are crucial for identifying specific food triggers and understanding individual tolerance levels.

3.3 Blood Tests

While dietary assessments and elimination diets are valuable tools, blood tests provide additional diagnostic information that can help confirm histamine intolerance.

DAO Levels

Diamine oxidase (DAO) is the primary enzyme responsible for breaking down ingested histamine. Measuring DAO levels can provide insight into histamine intolerance.

- Measuring DAO Activity:
- Blood tests can measure DAO activity levels. Low DAO levels can support a diagnosis of histamine intolerance.
- Factors such as genetic predisposition, intestinal damage, and certain medications can affect DAO levels.

- Interpreting Results:
- DAO levels should be interpreted alongside clinical symptoms and dietary assessments. A low DAO level alone does not confirm histamine intolerance but strengthens the diagnostic case when correlated with symptoms and dietary triggers.

Histamine Levels

Measuring plasma histamine levels can help determine if histamine intolerance is present.

- Histamine Concentration:
- Elevated histamine levels in the blood suggest that the body is not adequately breaking down histamine, leading to symptoms.
- Histamine levels can fluctuate based on dietary intake, stress, and other factors, so multiple measurements may be necessary.

- Relevance to Symptoms:
- Elevated histamine levels need to be considered in the context of symptoms and DAO activity to form a comprehensive diagnosis.

3.4 Differential Diagnosis

Histamine intolerance symptoms overlap with many other conditions, making differential diagnosis essential to rule out other potential causes.

Conditions that Mimic Histamine Intolerance

1. Allergies:

- Allergies can cause symptoms similar to histamine intolerance, such as hives, itching, nasal congestion, and respiratory issues.

- Skin prick tests, specific IgE testing, and patient history can help differentiate allergies from histamine intolerance.

2. Food Intolerances:

- Other food intolerances, such as lactose or gluten intolerance, can cause gastrointestinal symptoms like bloating, diarrhea, and stomach pain.

- Elimination diets and specific food intolerance tests can help identify these conditions.

3. Mast Cell Activation Syndrome (MCAS):

- MCAS is a condition where mast cells release excessive histamine and other chemicals, causing symptoms similar to histamine intolerance.

- Diagnosis involves measuring tryptase levels, assessing for other mast cell mediators, and considering patient history and symptoms.

3.5 Advanced Diagnostic Methods

Several advanced diagnostic methods are used to identify histamine intolerance, each with its own advantages and limitations.

Serum DAO Measurement

- Challenges and Considerations:

- Serum DAO levels can vary within the same individual over the course of the day, influenced by factors such as the time of day and recent food intake.

- DAO measurement should be used in conjunction with other diagnostic techniques rather than as a standalone test.

Histamine Challenge Test

- Purpose and Limitations:
- The histamine challenge test helps determine an individual's histamine tolerance threshold. However, measuring histamine levels in food accurately is challenging, and the test requires expert technical supervision.
- There are reports of this test inducing symptoms in healthy individuals, limiting its usefulness.

Histamine Levels in Feces

- Interference from Gut Bacteria:
- Measuring histamine levels in feces is proposed as a diagnostic method, but gut bacteria also produce histamine, obscuring the accuracy of this test.

Genetic Analysis

- Genetic Predisposition:

- Genetic analysis is gaining traction and can be useful when combined with other techniques. Certain single-nucleotide polymorphisms have been identified that predispose individuals to histamine intolerance.

- Genetic testing can be used in conjunction with other tests to confirm the diagnosis in susceptible individuals.

Diagnosing histamine intolerance requires a methodical and integrative approach, incorporating medical history, symptom tracking, dietary interventions, and specific blood tests. Differentiating histamine intolerance from other similar conditions is crucial for accurate diagnosis and effective treatment. By understanding and implementing these diagnostic strategies, healthcare providers can better identify histamine intolerance and help patients manage their symptoms effectively.

CHAPTER FOUR

Treatment and Management Options for Histamine Intolerance

Effectively managing histamine intolerance requires a comprehensive approach encompassing dietary modifications, supplements, and medications. Understanding and implementing these treatment strategies can significantly improve symptoms and enhance the quality of life for individuals suffering from this condition.

4.1 Dietary Modifications

Dietary modifications are the cornerstone of managing histamine intolerance. A low-histamine diet involves reducing the intake of foods that are high in histamine or that promote histamine release in the body. This dietary approach helps minimize the symptoms associated with histamine intolerance, such as headaches, digestive issues, skin reactions, and respiratory problems.

Overview of a Low-Histamine Diet

A low-histamine diet is not a one-size-fits-all solution; it requires personalization based on individual tolerance levels and symptom responses. The general principle is to avoid foods that are known to be high in histamine or that trigger histamine release. The primary focus is on steering clear of foods high in biogenic amines and histamine.

Foods to Avoid

Certain foods are notorious for their high histamine content or their ability to stimulate histamine release. Avoiding these foods is crucial for managing histamine intolerance:

- **Aged Cheeses:** Cheeses like Parmesan, Gouda, and Roquefort are high in histamine due to the aging process.
- **Cured and Processed Meats:** Salami, ham, sausages, and other processed meats contain high levels of histamine.
- **Fermented Foods and Beverages:** Sauerkraut, kimchi, soy sauce, vinegar, and alcoholic beverages like wine and beer have significant histamine content.
- **Certain Fish:** Fish like mackerel, sardines, tuna, and anchovies are prone to high histamine levels, especially when not fresh.
- **Vegetables:** Some vegetables, such as tomatoes, spinach, eggplants, and avocados, can contain higher levels of histamine.
- **Fruits:** Strawberries, bananas, pineapples, and citrus fruits can trigger histamine release.
- **Beverages:** Alcoholic drinks, especially red wine and champagne, as well as certain teas like black and green tea, can increase histamine levels.

- **Other Foods:** Chocolates, nuts, and some types of yeast and yeast-containing products should also be avoided.

Foods to Include

While the list of foods to avoid may seem extensive, there are plenty of low-histamine foods that can be safely included in the diet:

- **Fresh Meat and Poultry:** Freshly cooked, unprocessed meats like chicken, turkey, and lamb are low in histamine.
- **Fresh Fish:** Freshly caught and promptly cooked fish, such as salmon and cod, are generally low in histamine.
- **Fresh Vegetables:** Vegetables such as carrots, zucchini, bell peppers, and leafy greens (excluding spinach) are typically low in histamine.
- **Fruits:** Low-histamine fruits include apples, pears, and berries like blueberries and cranberries.

- **Grains:** Rice, oats, quinoa, and other gluten-free grains are safe options.
- **Dairy Alternatives:** Plant-based milks like almond milk, rice milk, and coconut milk are suitable substitutes for traditional dairy.
- **Herbs and Spices:** Fresh herbs like basil, parsley, and thyme, and spices like turmeric and ginger, are safe to use and can enhance the flavor of meals.
- **Other Foods:** Eggs, provided they are fresh, and certain oils like olive oil and coconut oil can be included in a low-histamine diet.

When employing this strategy, it's crucial to let patients who are histamine-intolerant know that certain food categories may be reintroduced in the future in specific amounts. Studies indicate that patients who benefit from this treatment plan ought to stick with it for a month or until their symptoms go away. Food is then progressively added back in. A low-dose histamine diet approach has been found to improve DAO levels in those who followed the diet, as well as ameliorate gastrointestinal, cutaneous, and other symptoms.

4.2 Supplements

In addition to dietary modifications, certain supplements can help manage histamine intolerance by supporting the body's ability to break down histamine or by replenishing nutrients that may be deficient.

DAO Supplements

Diamine oxidase (DAO) is the enzyme responsible for breaking down histamine in the digestive tract. For individuals with histamine intolerance, supplementing with DAO can help mitigate symptoms.

Numerous research studies have produced encouraging results regarding the use of exogenous DAO supplements. These supplements, usually derived from porcine sources, can be taken before meals to enhance the breakdown of dietary histamine. DAO supplementation can particularly benefit individuals with low endogenous DAO activity, helping to reduce symptoms like headaches, gastrointestinal distress, and skin reactions.

Komericki et al. assessed the effect of oral DAO supplementation on 39 patients who demonstrated symptoms of histamine intolerance. According to their findings, DAO supplementation led to a statistically significant improvement in symptoms when compared to a placebo. Similarly, Schnedl et al. found that taking DAO supplements considerably reduced the severity of all 22 symptoms related to histamine intolerance in a study involving 28 patients. Other studies, such as those by Manzotti et al., Yacoub et al., and Izquierdo-Casas et al., have also shown that DAO supplementation can improve symptoms like urticaria and headaches. However, while these studies show promising results, larger-scale research is necessary to validate the findings.

Vitamins and Minerals

Certain vitamins and minerals play crucial roles in histamine metabolism and can support overall health in individuals with histamine intolerance:

- **Vitamin C:** Acts as a natural antihistamine by breaking down histamine. Foods rich in vitamin C, such as bell peppers, broccoli, and kiwi, should be included in the diet.
- **Vitamin B6:** A cofactor in the activity of DAO and can help enhance its function. Sources of vitamin B6 include chicken, turkey, chickpeas, and bananas. Supplementation may be necessary for some individuals.
- **Magnesium:** Plays a role in stabilizing mast cells, which release histamine. Leafy green vegetables, nuts, seeds, and whole grains are good dietary sources of magnesium.
- Quercetin: A flavonoid with natural antihistamine properties. Foods high in

quercetin include onions, apples, and capers. Quercetin supplements are also available.

4.3 Medications

When dietary modifications and supplements are insufficient to control symptoms, medications can be used to manage histamine intolerance. These medications work by blocking histamine receptors or reducing histamine release.

Antihistamines

Antihistamines are the most commonly used medications to manage symptoms of histamine intolerance. They work by blocking the action of histamine at its receptors.

- **H1 Antihistamines:** Medications such as cetirizine, loratadine, and diphenhydramine are effective in treating symptoms like itching, hives, and nasal congestion. These medications are available over-the-counter and by prescription, and they provide quick relief from acute symptoms.

- H2 Antihistamines: Medications such as ranitidine and famotidine reduce stomach acid production and can help alleviate gastrointestinal symptoms associated with histamine intolerance, such as acid reflux and indigestion.

Other Medications

In addition to antihistamines, other medications can help manage the symptoms of histamine intolerance:

- Mast Cell Stabilizers: Medications like cromolyn sodium can stabilize mast cells, preventing them from releasing histamine and other inflammatory mediators. These medications are often used in chronic cases where mast cell activation is a significant contributor to symptoms.

- Probiotics: Certain probiotics, such as Lactobacillus rhamnosus and Bifidobacterium longum, can help modulate the gut microbiota and reduce histamine production in the gut. Regular use of probiotics can support gut health and potentially reduce the severity of histamine intolerance symptoms.

- Anti-inflammatory Drugs: Nonsteroidal anti-inflammatory drugs (NSAIDs) like ibuprofen can help manage inflammation and pain associated with histamine intolerance. However, some individuals with histamine intolerance may be sensitive to NSAIDs, so these should be used with caution and under medical supervision.

Managing histamine intolerance involves a multifaceted approach, including dietary modifications, supplements, and medications. By understanding and implementing these treatment strategies, individuals with histamine intolerance can significantly reduce their symptoms and improve their overall quality of life. Collaboration with healthcare providers, including dietitians and physicians, is essential to tailor treatment plans to individual needs and ensure the most effective management of this complex condition.

CHAPTER FIVE

Recovery from Histamine Intolerance

Recovering from histamine intolerance can be a complex journey that requires time, patience, and consistent effort. The process involves not only managing and alleviating symptoms but also understanding the underlying causes and adjusting one's lifestyle to support long-term health. This chapter explores the timeline of recovery, monitoring progress, and essential strategies to ensure effective management of histamine intolerance.

5.1 Timeline of Recovery

Short-Term vs. Long-Term Expectations

Recovery from histamine intolerance is highly individual and can vary greatly from one person to another. Factors such as the severity of symptoms, underlying health conditions, and adherence to treatment plans all play a role in determining the recovery timeline.

Short-Term Expectations:
In the initial phase of treatment, typically the first month, the primary goal is symptom management and stabilization. During this period, individuals usually experience a noticeable reduction in acute symptoms, such as headaches, gastrointestinal distress, and skin reactions, through dietary modifications and the use of supplements or medications.

- **Dietary Changes:** Adopting a low-histamine diet often brings about significant improvement in symptoms within a few days to weeks. Eliminating high-histamine foods can quickly reduce the body's histamine load, leading to a decrease in symptom severity.

- **Supplements:** Introducing supplements like diamine oxidase (DAO) and essential vitamins can enhance the body's ability to metabolize histamine, further alleviating symptoms. Many individuals report feeling better within a few weeks of starting these supplements.

- Medications: For those with severe symptoms, medications such as antihistamines can provide rapid relief. These are typically used in the short term to control acute reactions while other long-term strategies are implemented.

Long-Term Expectations:

Long-term recovery involves a more comprehensive approach aimed at addressing the root causes of histamine intolerance and preventing recurrence. This phase can span several months to years and focuses on maintaining symptom control, healing the gut, and ensuring nutritional balance.

- **Gradual Reintroduction of Foods:** After the initial strict adherence to a low-histamine diet, individuals may begin to slowly reintroduce foods to identify specific triggers. This process is crucial for creating a sustainable and varied diet.

- **Gut Health:** Long-term recovery often includes strategies to improve gut health, such as incorporating probiotics, prebiotics, and anti-inflammatory foods. A healthy gut microbiome can enhance histamine metabolism and reduce overall histamine levels.

- **Lifestyle Adjustments:** Stress management, regular exercise, and adequate sleep are vital components of long-term recovery. These lifestyle factors can influence histamine levels and overall immune function.

- **Continuous Monitoring:** Long-term management requires ongoing monitoring of symptoms and dietary intake to make necessary adjustments and prevent relapse.

While short-term recovery focuses on immediate symptom relief, long-term recovery aims to establish a balanced and resilient state of health, minimizing the likelihood of future histamine-related issues.

5.2 Monitoring Progress

Effective management and recovery from histamine intolerance require diligent monitoring of symptoms and dietary intake. Keeping a symptom and food diary, along with regular medical check-ups, are essential tools in tracking progress and making informed adjustments to the treatment plan.

Keeping a Symptom and Food Diary

A symptom and food diary is a powerful tool for identifying patterns and correlations between diet, lifestyle factors, and symptoms. This practice helps in fine-tuning the dietary plan and understanding individual triggers.

- **Daily Entries:** Record all meals, snacks, beverages, and supplements consumed each day. Include details such as portion sizes, ingredients, and preparation methods. Note any deviations from the prescribed low-histamine diet.

- **Symptom Tracking:** Document any symptoms experienced, including their severity, duration, and onset time relative to food intake. Common symptoms to track include headaches, digestive issues, skin reactions, respiratory problems, and fatigue.

- **Lifestyle Factors:** Include notes on stress levels, physical activity, sleep quality, and any other relevant lifestyle factors. These can influence histamine levels and symptom severity.

- **Pattern Identification:** Over time, review the diary to identify patterns and specific triggers. For example, certain foods or combinations of foods may consistently lead to symptoms, while others may be well-tolerated.

- **Adjustment and Adaptation:** Use the information gathered to make informed decisions about dietary adjustments and lifestyle changes. For instance, if a particular food consistently causes symptoms, it may need to be eliminated or restricted.

Maintaining a detailed symptom and food diary can provide valuable insights that facilitate a more personalized and effective approach to managing histamine intolerance.

Regular Medical Check-Ups

Regular medical check-ups are crucial for monitoring overall health and the effectiveness of the treatment plan. These check-ups provide an opportunity for healthcare professionals to assess progress, address any concerns, and make necessary adjustments.

- **Initial Assessment:** An initial comprehensive assessment by a healthcare provider, preferably one with experience in histamine intolerance, is essential. This assessment should include a detailed medical history, dietary habits, symptom evaluation, and any relevant laboratory tests.

- **Follow-Up Visits:** Schedule regular follow-up visits to track progress and make adjustments to the treatment plan. The frequency of these visits may vary depending on the severity of symptoms and the individual's response to treatment.

- **Laboratory Tests:** Periodic laboratory tests may be necessary to monitor specific markers, such as DAO activity, histamine levels, nutrient deficiencies, and gut health indicators. These tests provide objective data to support treatment decisions.

- **Medication Review:** For individuals using medications such as antihistamines or DAO supplements, regular review and adjustment of dosages may be needed to ensure optimal efficacy and minimize potential side effects.

- **Comprehensive Care:** Collaboration with a multidisciplinary team, including dietitians, gastroenterologists, and allergists, can provide comprehensive care and support. This team approach ensures that all aspects of histamine intolerance are addressed.

Regular medical check-ups and ongoing communication with healthcare providers are essential components of a successful recovery plan. These check-ups allow for timely interventions and adjustments, ensuring that the treatment strategy remains effective and responsive to the individual's needs.

Recovery from histamine intolerance is a multifaceted and ongoing process that requires commitment and collaboration between patients and healthcare providers. By understanding the timeline of recovery, keeping a detailed symptom and food diary, and maintaining regular medical check-ups, individuals can effectively manage their condition and improve their quality of life. This holistic approach not only addresses immediate symptoms but also fosters long-term health and resilience, paving the way for sustained well-being.

CHAPTER SIX

Diet Plan for Histamine Intolerance

Developing a diet plan for histamine intolerance requires careful consideration of which foods to avoid and which to include. A well-structured approach not only alleviates symptoms but also ensures nutritional adequacy and enjoyment of meals. This chapter provides detailed guidelines on foods to avoid, safe food options, meal planning tips, and delicious recipes to make the journey enjoyable and effective.

6.1 Foods to Avoid

Managing histamine intolerance begins with eliminating foods that are high in histamine or act as histamine liberators. These foods can exacerbate symptoms and hinder recovery.

High-Histamine Foods

High-histamine foods are those that naturally contain significant amounts of histamine due to their aging, fermentation, or spoilage. Avoiding these foods is crucial to managing symptoms.

- **Aged Cheeses:** Parmesan, Gouda, Roquefort, and other aged cheeses accumulate histamine during the aging process.
- **Cured and Processed Meats:** Salami, ham, sausages, and other cured meats are high in histamine.
- **Fermented Foods and Beverages:** Sauerkraut, kimchi, soy sauce, vinegar, and alcoholic beverages like wine and beer are rich in histamine.
- **Certain Fish:** Fish such as mackerel, sardines, tuna, and anchovies can develop high histamine levels, especially if not fresh.

- **Certain Vegetables:** Tomatoes, spinach, eggplants, and avocados contain higher levels of histamine.
- **Certain Fruits:** Strawberries, bananas, pineapples, and citrus fruits can trigger histamine release.
- **Other Foods:** Chocolates, nuts, and some yeast-containing products should also be avoided.

Histamine Liberators

Histamine liberators are foods that can trigger the release of histamine stored in the body's cells, even if they do not contain high levels of histamine themselves.

- **Citrus Fruits:** Oranges, lemons, limes, and grapefruits can prompt histamine release.
- **Certain Additives:** Food colorings, preservatives, and other additives can act as histamine liberators.

- **Alcohol:** Alcohol, particularly red wine and beer, can cause histamine release and should be avoided.

6.2 Low-Histamine Foods

To maintain a balanced and enjoyable diet while managing histamine intolerance, focus on foods that are low in histamine and unlikely to trigger histamine release.

Safe Food Options

While the list of foods to avoid may seem extensive, there are plenty of low-histamine foods that can be safely included in your diet.

- **Fresh Meat and Poultry:** Freshly cooked, unprocessed meats like chicken, turkey, and lamb are low in histamine.
- **Fresh Fish:** Freshly caught and promptly cooked fish, such as salmon and cod, are generally low in histamine.

- **Fresh Vegetables:** Vegetables such as carrots, zucchini, bell peppers, and leafy greens (excluding spinach) are typically low in histamine.
- **Fruits:** Low-histamine fruits include apples, pears, and berries like blueberries and cranberries.
- **Grains:** Rice, oats, quinoa, and other gluten-free grains are safe options.
- **Dairy Alternatives:** Plant-based milks like almond milk, rice milk, and coconut milk are suitable substitutes for traditional dairy.
- **Herbs and Spices:** Fresh herbs like basil, parsley, and thyme, and spices like turmeric and ginger, are safe to use and can enhance the flavor of meals.
- **Other Foods:** Eggs (provided they are fresh) and certain oils like olive oil and coconut oil can be included in a low-histamine diet.

6.3 Meal Planning Tips

Creating balanced meals that are both nutritious and enjoyable is key to adhering to a low-histamine diet. Here are some tips to help you plan effectively and sample meal plans to get you started.

Creating Balanced Meals

Balance and variety are essential to ensuring your diet remains enjoyable and nutritionally adequate.

- **Protein:** Include fresh, unprocessed meats, poultry, or fish in each meal.
- **Carbohydrates:** Incorporate low-histamine grains such as rice, quinoa, or oats.
- **Fruits and Vegetables:** Aim for a variety of fresh vegetables and low-histamine fruits to provide essential vitamins and minerals.
- **Healthy Fats:** Use safe oils like olive oil and coconut oil, and include nuts and seeds that are low in histamine.
- **Herbs and Spices:** Enhance flavors with safe herbs and spices to make meals more enjoyable.

Sample Meal Plans

Here are a few sample meal plans to illustrate how you can create delicious, low-histamine meals.

Day 1:
- Breakfast: Oatmeal with blueberries and a drizzle of honey.
- Lunch: Grilled chicken salad with mixed greens, carrots, cucumbers, and olive oil dressing.
- Dinner: Baked salmon with quinoa and steamed zucchini.
- Snack: Sliced apple with almond butter.

Day 2:
- Breakfast: Smoothie with almond milk, spinach, and pear.
- Lunch: Turkey and avocado wrap with a side of fresh carrot sticks.
- Dinner: Stir-fried beef with bell peppers and broccoli over brown rice.
- Snack: Fresh berries with coconut yogurt.

Day 3:
- Breakfast: Scrambled eggs with fresh herbs and a side of quinoa.
- Lunch: Cod fillet with sweet potato mash and steamed green beans.
- Dinner: Chicken and vegetable soup with a side of rice cakes.
- Snack: Sliced cucumber with hummus.

6.4 Recipes

To make meal planning easier and more enjoyable, here are some low-histamine recipes for breakfast, lunch, dinner, and snacks.

Breakfast

Oatmeal with Blueberries and Honey
- Ingredients:
  - 1 cup oats
  - 2 cups water or almond milk
  - 1 cup fresh blueberries
  - 1 tbsp honey

  - 1 tsp cinnamon

- **Instructions:**
1. Bring water or almond milk to a boil.
2. Add oats and reduce heat to a simmer. Cook for about 5 minutes, stirring occasionally.
3. Stir in blueberries, honey, and cinnamon.
4. Serve warm and enjoy.

Lunch

Grilled Chicken Salad
- Ingredients:
  - 1 grilled chicken breast, sliced
  - 2 cups mixed greens
  - 1 carrot, shredded
  - 1 cucumber, sliced
  - 2 tbsp olive oil
  - 1 tbsp apple cider vinegar
  - Salt and pepper to taste

- **Instructions:**

1. In a large bowl, combine mixed greens, carrot, and cucumber.

2. Top with sliced grilled chicken.

3. In a small bowl, whisk together olive oil, vinegar, salt, and pepper.

4. Drizzle dressing over salad and toss to combine.

5. Serve immediately.

Dinner

Baked Salmon with Quinoa and Zucchini
- Ingredients:
  - 1 salmon fillet
  - 1 cup quinoa
  - 2 cups water
  - 1 zucchini, sliced
  - 2 tbsp olive oil
  - 1 lemon, sliced
  - Salt and pepper to taste

- Instructions:
1. Preheat oven to 375°F (190°C).

2. Place salmon on a baking sheet, drizzle with olive oil, and season with salt, pepper, and lemon slices.

3. Bake for 20 minutes or until salmon is cooked through.

4. Meanwhile, bring water to a boil, add quinoa, and reduce heat. Simmer for 15 minutes or until water is absorbed.

5. In a skillet, sauté zucchini slices in olive oil until tender.

6. Serve salmon with quinoa and sautéed zucchini on the side.

Snacks

Sliced Apple with Almond Butter
- Ingredients:
  - 1 apple, sliced
  - 2 tbsp almond butter
- Instructions:
  1. Slice apple into thin wedges.
  2. Serve with almond butter for dipping.
  3. Enjoy as a quick and nutritious snack.

Cucumber and Hummus

- Ingredients:
  - 1 cucumber, sliced
    - 1/2 cup homemade hummus (blend chickpeas, tahini, olive oil, lemon juice, and garlic)
- Instructions:
  1. Slice cucumber into rounds.
  2. Serve with hummus for dipping.
  3. Enjoy as a refreshing and healthy snack.

Creating a diet plan for histamine intolerance involves careful selection of foods to avoid and include, balanced meal planning, and incorporating delicious, low-histamine recipes. By following these guidelines, you can manage your histamine intolerance effectively while enjoying a varied and nutritious diet. This approach not only alleviates symptoms but also supports long-term health and well-being.

CHAPTER SEVEN

Long-Term Management and Living with Histamine Intolerance

Living with histamine intolerance involves more than just dietary changes; it requires a comprehensive approach to managing symptoms, adapting lifestyle habits, and finding psychological and emotional support. This chapter talks about the long-term strategies for managing histamine intolerance, coping with the emotional impact, and navigating social situations like dining out.

7.1 Monitoring and Adjusting Diet and Lifestyle

Adapting to Changes in Tolerance

Histamine intolerance is a dynamic condition, meaning that an individual's tolerance to histamine can change over time. Long-term management involves regularly monitoring and adjusting diet and lifestyle to accommodate these changes.

1. Keeping a Food and Symptom Diary:

- **Track Everything:** Documenting daily food intake and symptoms helps identify patterns and trigger foods.
- **Regular Reviews:** Periodically reviewing the diary with a healthcare provider can provide

insights into tolerance levels and necessary adjustments.

- **Flexibility:** Be prepared to modify the diet based on seasonal changes, stress levels, and other factors that might affect histamine levels.

2. Reintroducing Foods:

- **Gradual Process:** Reintroduce potentially problematic foods one at a time in small amounts to gauge tolerance.
- **Observe and Record:** Monitor symptoms carefully after reintroducing each food. Note any adverse reactions and adjust accordingly.
- **Rotational Diet:** Consider a rotational diet, where foods are consumed on a rotating basis to prevent overexposure to potential triggers.

3. Lifestyle Adjustments:

- **Stress Management:** High stress can increase histamine levels. Incorporate stress-reducing activities like yoga, meditation, and regular exercise.

- **Sleep Hygiene:** Ensure adequate and quality sleep, as poor sleep can exacerbate symptoms.
- **Environmental Factors:** Be mindful of other histamine triggers such as pollen, dust, and pet dander. Using air purifiers and maintaining a clean living environment can help.

7.2 Psychological and Emotional Support

Living with histamine intolerance can be emotionally challenging. It's essential to address the psychological impact and find effective coping strategies and support systems.

Coping Strategies

1. Education and Awareness:
- **Knowledge is Power:** Understanding the condition thoroughly can alleviate fear and uncertainty. Stay informed about new research and treatment options.
- **Empowerment:** Being knowledgeable enables you to make informed decisions about diet and lifestyle adjustments.

2. Mindfulness and Relaxation Techniques:
- **Mindfulness Practices:** Techniques such as meditation and deep breathing can help manage stress and anxiety.
- **Relaxation:** Activities like reading, listening to music, and spending time in nature can provide relaxation and mental clarity.

3. Cognitive Behavioral Therapy (CBT):
- **Professional Help:** Working with a therapist can help develop effective coping mechanisms and strategies to manage anxiety and depression associated with chronic illness.
- **Positive Thinking:** CBT focuses on changing negative thought patterns and fostering a positive mindset.

Support Groups and Resources

1. Finding Community:
- **Support Groups:** Joining support groups, either in-person or online, can provide a sense of community and shared experience. Platforms

like Facebook, Reddit, and specialized forums offer valuable resources and peer support.

- **Local Groups:** Check for local support groups or meetups through hospitals, clinics, or community centers.

2. Professional Support:

- **Dietitians and Nutritionists:** Regular consultations with professionals who specialize in histamine intolerance can help manage the condition effectively.

- **Mental Health Professionals:** Psychologists and counselors can assist in dealing with the emotional burden of the condition.

3. Educational Resources:

- **Books and Articles:** Numerous books and articles are available that provide comprehensive information about histamine intolerance.

- **Websites and Blogs:** Reputable websites and blogs often feature articles, recipes, and tips for managing the condition.

7.3 Tips for Eating Out

Managing histamine intolerance can be particularly challenging in social situations and restaurants. However, with some planning and awareness, you can enjoy dining out while keeping symptoms at bay.

Managing Histamine Intolerance in Social Situations and Restaurants

1. Research Ahead:
- **Restaurant Research:** Look for restaurants that offer flexible menu options and are willing to accommodate dietary restrictions. Many establishments now post their menus online, making it easier to plan ahead.
- **Special Requests:** Don't hesitate to call ahead and inquire if the restaurant can accommodate your needs.

2. Communicating with Staff:

- **Clear Communication:** Politely inform the server or chef about your dietary restrictions. Be specific about what you need to avoid and why.
- **Simplified Orders:** Opt for simple dishes with fresh ingredients. Avoid complex dishes that may contain hidden histamine-rich components.

3. Menu Choices:
- **Safe Options:** Stick to safe, low-histamine foods such as fresh salads (without tomatoes and aged dressings), grilled chicken or fish, and steamed vegetables.
- **Substitutions:** Request substitutions when necessary, such as replacing dressings with olive oil and lemon, or choosing plain sides instead of seasoned ones.

4. Emergency Preparations:
- **Bring Snacks:** Carry safe snacks like nuts or fruit in case the restaurant cannot accommodate your needs.

- **Medication:** Always have antihistamines or other prescribed medications on hand in case of accidental exposure.

5. Social Gatherings:

- **Host's Awareness:** Inform the host of your dietary needs well in advance if attending a gathering. Offer to bring a dish that you can safely eat.

- **Eat Before:** Consider eating a small meal before attending an event to ensure you're not overly hungry and tempted to eat unsuitable foods.

Long-term management of histamine intolerance requires a proactive and flexible approach to diet and lifestyle. By regularly monitoring symptoms and adjusting dietary intake, seeking psychological and emotional support, and mastering the art of dining out, individuals can lead a fulfilling life despite their condition. Building a strong support system, staying informed, and embracing adaptive strategies are key to managing histamine intolerance effectively and enjoying life to the fullest.

Conclusion

Summary of Key Points

Histamine intolerance is a complex condition that affects many people worldwide, often causing a range of symptoms that can significantly impact daily life. Managing this condition effectively requires a multifaceted approach that includes dietary modifications, supplements, medications, and lifestyle adjustments.

Understanding Histamine Intolerance: At its core, histamine intolerance results from an imbalance between the amount of histamine ingested or produced in the body and the ability to break it down, primarily due to a deficiency in the enzyme diamine oxidase (DAO).

Dietary Modifications: One of the most effective strategies for managing histamine intolerance is adhering to a low-histamine diet. This involves avoiding high-histamine foods like aged cheeses, cured meats, and fermented products, as well as histamine liberators that trigger the release of histamine in the body. Instead, focusing on fresh, unprocessed foods such as fresh meat, poultry, certain vegetables, and low-histamine fruits can help mitigate symptoms.

Supplementation: DAO supplements can be particularly beneficial for individuals with low endogenous DAO activity. Additionally, vitamins and minerals such as vitamin C, vitamin B6, magnesium, and quercetin play crucial roles in histamine metabolism and can support overall health.

Medications: When dietary changes and supplements are insufficient, medications like antihistamines and mast cell stabilizers can be used to manage symptoms. Antihistamines block the action of histamine at its receptors, providing quick relief, while mast cell stabilizers prevent the release of histamine and other inflammatory mediators.

Monitoring and Adjusting: Long-term management of histamine intolerance involves regular monitoring and adjustments based on changes in tolerance. Keeping a food and symptom diary, reintroducing foods gradually, and making lifestyle adjustments such as stress management and improving sleep hygiene are crucial components of this strategy.

Psychological and Emotional Support: The psychological impact of living with histamine intolerance can be significant. Effective coping strategies include mindfulness and relaxation techniques, cognitive behavioral therapy (CBT), and seeking support from community groups and mental health professionals.

Dining Out: Navigating social situations and dining out requires careful planning and communication. Researching restaurants, informing staff about dietary restrictions, opting for simple dishes, and carrying safe snacks and medications can help manage the condition in social settings.

Future Directions in Research

While current management strategies for histamine intolerance focus on dietary and lifestyle adjustments, supplementation, and medications, ongoing research continues to explore emerging treatments and diagnostic tools that could revolutionize the approach to this condition.

Emerging Treatments

1. Advanced DAO Supplements:
- **New Formulations:** Research is underway to develop more effective DAO supplements with enhanced absorption and bioavailability. These new formulations aim to improve the efficiency of histamine breakdown in the digestive tract, providing better symptom control.

- **Plant-Based DAO:** Exploring plant-based sources of DAO offers a potential alternative for individuals who are unable to use animal-derived supplements.

2. Probiotic Therapy:

- **Gut Microbiota Modulation:** The gut microbiota plays a significant role in histamine metabolism. Probiotics like Lactobacillus rhamnosus and Bifidobacterium longum have shown promise in modulating gut microbiota and reducing histamine production. Future research could lead to the development of targeted probiotic therapies specifically designed to manage histamine intolerance.

3. Enzyme Replacement Therapy:

- **Synthetic Enzymes:** Advances in biotechnology are paving the way for synthetic enzyme replacement therapies. By providing a consistent supply of histamine-degrading enzymes, this approach could offer a more permanent solution for individuals with DAO deficiency.

4. Histamine Receptor Modulators:

- **Selective Antagonists:** Developing selective histamine receptor modulators that target specific histamine receptors (e.g., H1, H2, H3, H4) could offer more precise and effective symptom relief with fewer side effects compared to broad-spectrum antihistamines.

Diagnostic Tools

1. Biomarker Identification:

- **Genetic Markers:** Identifying genetic markers associated with DAO deficiency and histamine intolerance can help in early diagnosis and personalized treatment plans. Genetic testing could become a routine part of diagnosing histamine intolerance, allowing for more tailored interventions.

- **Serum Biomarkers:** Research is focused on identifying specific serum biomarkers that correlate with histamine intolerance. These biomarkers could provide a non-invasive and accurate method for diagnosing the condition and monitoring treatment efficacy.

2. Advanced Imaging Techniques:

- Gut Imaging: Advanced imaging techniques, such as functional MRI and PET scans, are being explored to assess gut health and histamine metabolism. These imaging tools could provide valuable insights into the underlying mechanisms of histamine intolerance and guide treatment strategies.

3. Wearable Technology:

- Real-Time Monitoring: Wearable devices equipped with sensors to monitor histamine levels and other relevant biomarkers in real-time are an exciting development. These devices could alert individuals to potential histamine spikes, allowing for immediate intervention and better symptom management.

4. Machine Learning and AI:

- Predictive Models: Machine learning and artificial intelligence are being utilized to develop predictive models for histamine intolerance. By analyzing large datasets, these models can identify patterns and predict individual responses to various treatments, leading to more personalized and effective management plans.

The journey of managing histamine intolerance is multifaceted, requiring a combination of dietary modifications, lifestyle adjustments, and medical interventions. As our understanding of this condition deepens, ongoing research continues to offer hope for more effective treatments and diagnostic tools. By staying informed about emerging therapies and leveraging advanced diagnostic techniques, individuals with histamine intolerance can look forward to improved quality of life and better symptom management in the future.

Embracing a proactive and informed approach, along with seeking support from healthcare professionals and community resources, can empower individuals to live well with histamine intolerance. As science progresses, the future holds promising advancements that will undoubtedly enhance our ability to diagnose, treat, and manage this complex condition.